Yoga
on the
Edge

The
Step-by-Step
Chair Yoga
Picture Book
for
Teachers
and Students

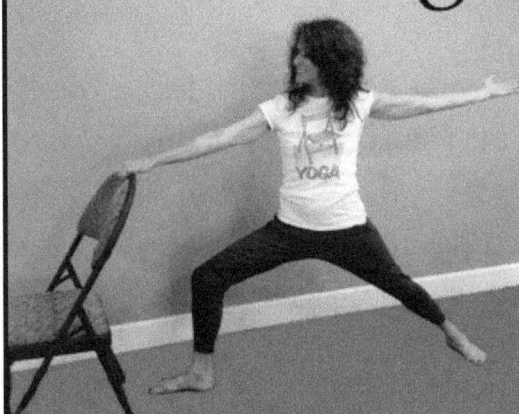

ANNETTE
WERTMAN

Yoga on the Edge
The Step-by-Step Chair Yoga Picture Book for Teachers and Students

ISBN: 978-1500501754

Photographs by Annette Wertman and friends
Cover design by Kathrin Lake

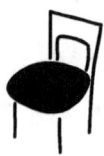

Table of Contents

INTRODUCTION

A few years ago now, my son suggested that if I took up yoga, it might reduce my stress level. I certainly did not plan to start another career when I walked into my first yoga class at the age of 55. But, it did not take long for me to notice that not only did I feel less stressed but also stronger and more flexible. After a couple years of dedicated practice, I wanted to share this revelation with others, so I committed to attaining a certification to teach yoga. That was the start.

One day, while visiting the Jewish Community Centre to observe a yoga class for seniors, I was mistakenly interviewed for the "Chair Yoga" instructor position. Since I was certified to teach yoga, combined with my experience as a music therapist with older adults, I was certainly qualified to fill the position. Fate having taken a hand, I walked away with the job.

Since then, I have continued to lead Chair Yoga classes at the Jewish Community Centre and other facilities. I even offer a unique Friday class called "Shabbat Yoga," incorporating some Jewish traditions of the Sabbath. Both practices share a focus on community, tolerance, peace and compassion. I soon realized that I was bringing yoga to a mature demographic, many of whom had never experienced yoga before. Together we have modified and adapted many yoga asanas (poses), to include a "chair" instead of the traditional yoga mat. Chair Yoga now becomes safe and accessible to almost anyone!

I received a Master of Arts degree in Gerontology from Simon Fraser University in December 2013. My thesis was titled, "Yoga and the Older Adult: An Exploratory Study." The research results convinced me of the health benefits of a regular, dedicated yoga practice. I co-teach a 35- hour Chair Yoga Teacher Training course at Semperviva Yoga, Vancouver, BC. Certified Chair Yoga teachers are needed.

My yoga class participants, and the students in my teacher training courses, asked for a guidebook they could use to practice from at home or when travelling. It is because of them that I compiled this simple, easy to follow Chair Yoga manual. *Yoga on the Edge* refers to sitting on the edge of the chair, as well as breaking new ground in Yoga practices for everyone.

I want to thank the people who gave me their permission to use their photographs.

Namaste,

Annette Wertman
http://agelessyoga.ca.

GUIDELINES

1. Tell people, most importantly your health care practitioner, that you are practicing yoga.
2. Use a sturdy, stable straight back chair, with a secure seat.
3. Practice in a warm quiet place, without external distractions.
4. Never force a movement or struggle with a pose.
5. Listen to your body and only repeat movements as you are comfortable.
6. Breathe consciously with each movement.

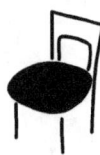

CHAIR ASANA

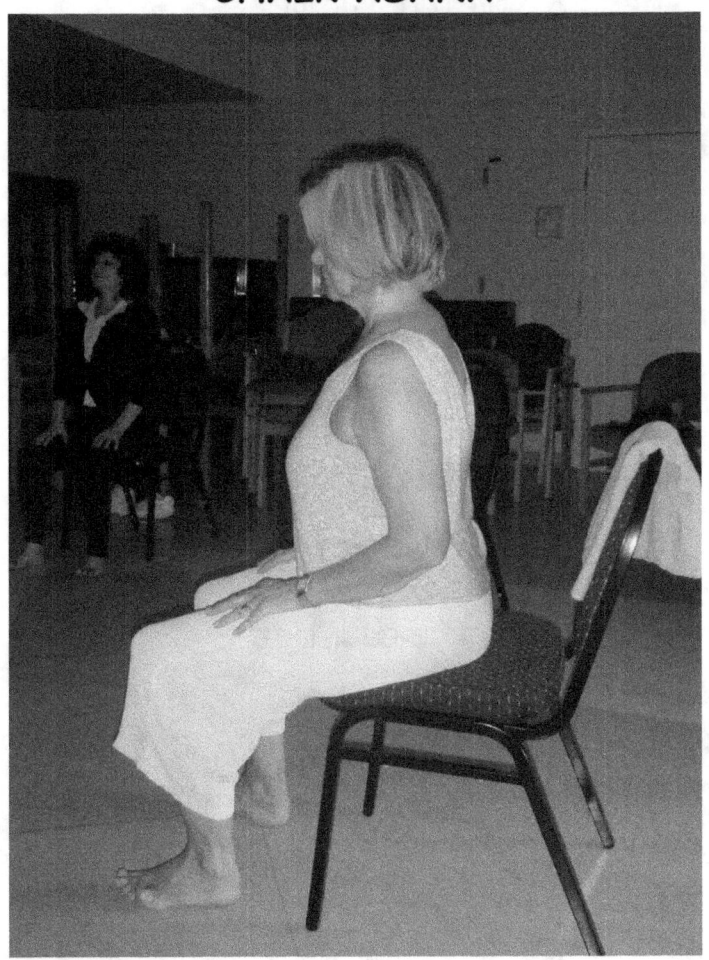

CHAIR POSTURE

1. Sit tall, on the edge of your seat, in a sturdy, stable chair.
2. Bare feet, flat on the floor, feet underneath your knees.
3. Knees and feet two fists distance apart.
4. Pull in your belly.

WARM-UPS

Rotate, bend & stretch, wiggle:

1. Ankles & Toes
2. Hips & Knees & Legs
3. Head & Neck & Eyes
4. Shoulders
5. Fingers & Hands & Arms
6. Spine

OM-GRATITUDE-MEDITATION

1. Gently close your eyes.
2. Slowly *inhale* to the count of 4.
   Exhale chanting OM.
3. Chant: ***"May all beings be happy & free and may the happiness and freedom of my life contribute in some way to the happiness and freedom of all beings"***
   (Lokah Samasta Sukino Bavantu)
4. Sit in stillness for a few minutes. Focus on your breath.
5. Breathe deeper, smoother, and slower with each breath.

PRANAYAMA

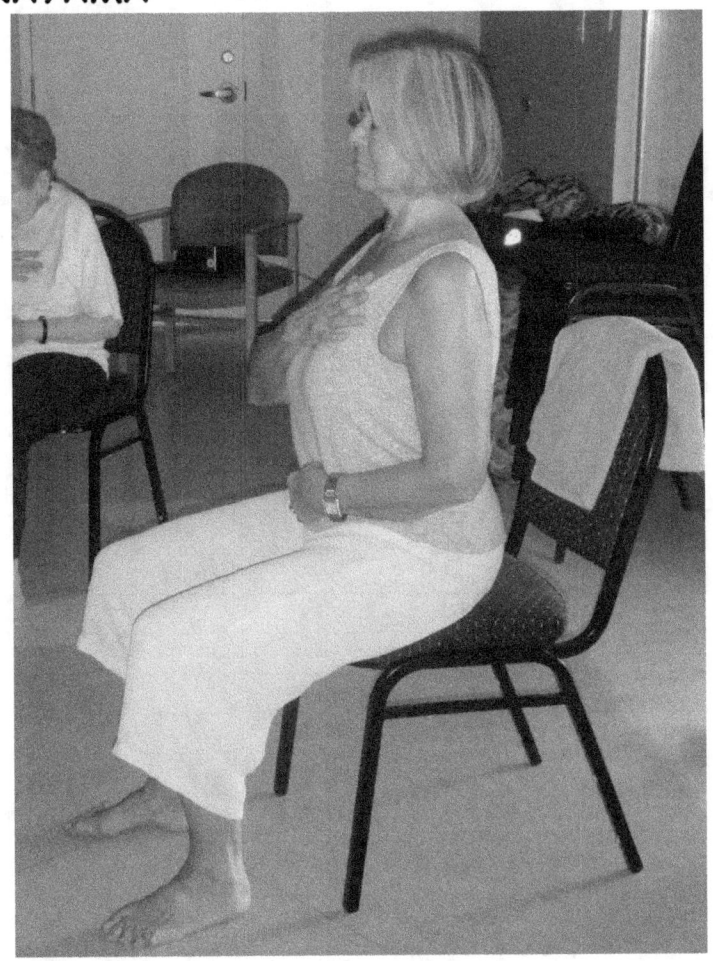

FEEL YOUR BREATHING:

1. Hand on chest
2. Hand on belly
3. Hands on rib cage

ASANAS: POSTURES
SEQUENCE #1 Seated
#1: ANGEL BREATH

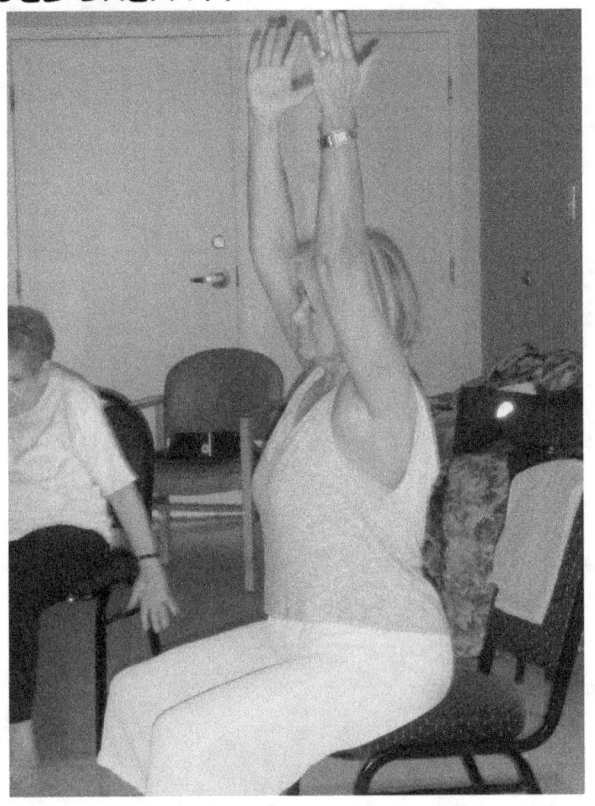

1. Sit tall at the edge of the chair.
2. Press feet firmly into the floor and relax your shoulders.
3. *Inhale* and slowly and raise your arms above your head.
4. Reach up.
5. *Exhale* and slowly bring your arms down. Repeat a few times.

#2: HALF MOON - ARDHA CHANDRASANA

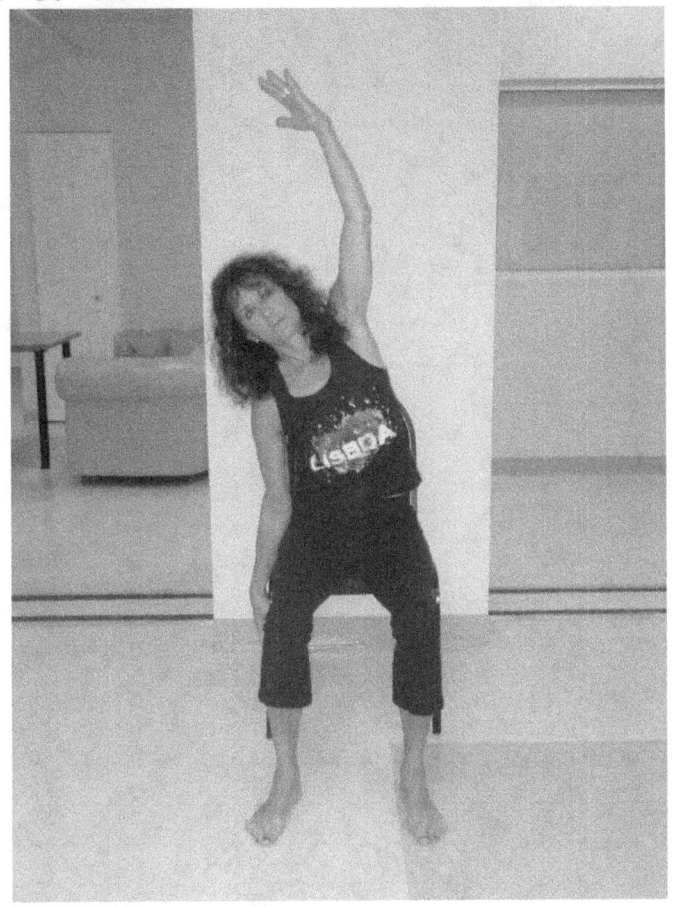

1. *Inhale* sitting tall.
2. Slowly *exhale* as you stretch your right hand up and over your head.
3. *Inhale* as you return to a straight spine.
4. Repeat same side 2 or 3 more times.
5. Switch sides.

#3: CAT/COW - MARJARIASANA

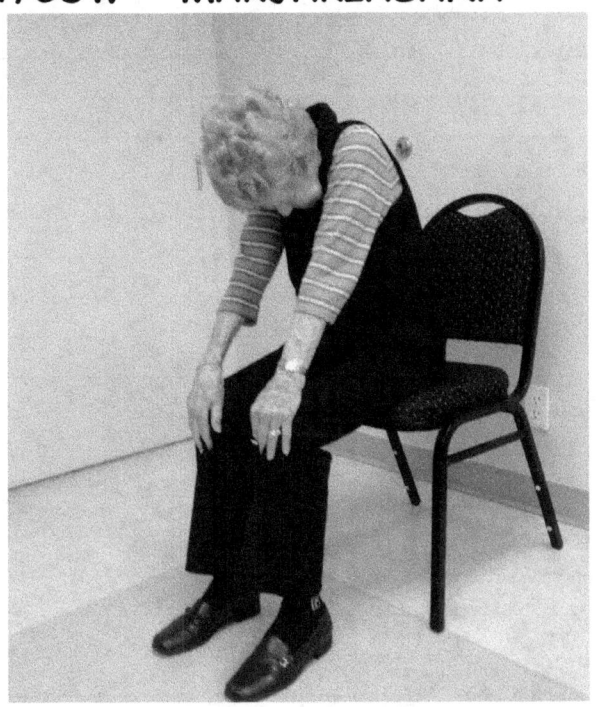

1. Palms down, spread fingers on knees with straight arms.
2. As you *inhale* slowly, arch your back, look up, chin up, puff out your chest and feel your shoulder blades coming together down on your back.
3. Experience the sensation of expanding your rib cage up and out.
4. As you slowly *exhale*, pull your belly button towards your spine, round your back and bring your chin to your chest.
5. Do this movement (asana) 3 to 5 times.

#4: SPINAL TWIST- MATSYENDRASANA

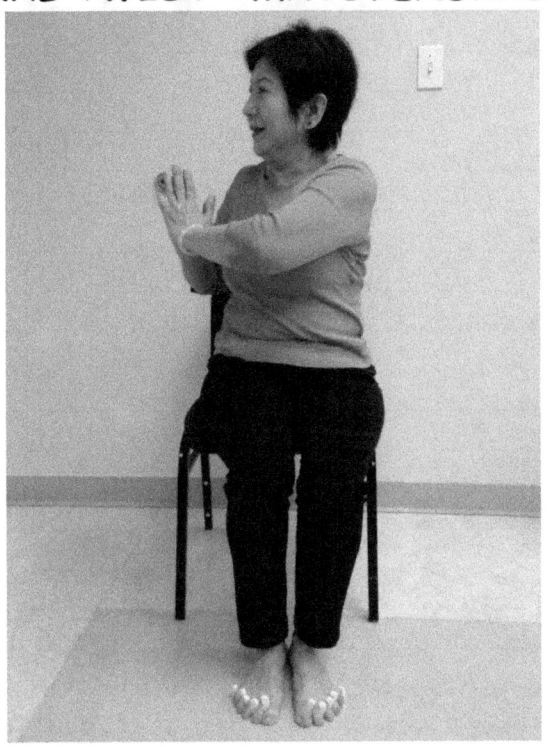

1. Palms together at your heart, gently pressing fingertips and wrists together, elbows up with forearms parallel to the ground.
2. *Inhale* to lengthen your spine, as you slowly *exhale* turn to the right, keeping your head in line with your hands.
3. *Inhale* deeply in this twisted position, *exhaling* as you slowly turn back to center.
4. Repeat this movement 3 to 5 times.
5. Now repeat this twist to the left 3 to 5 times.

#5: FORWARD BEND – PACHIMOTTANASANA

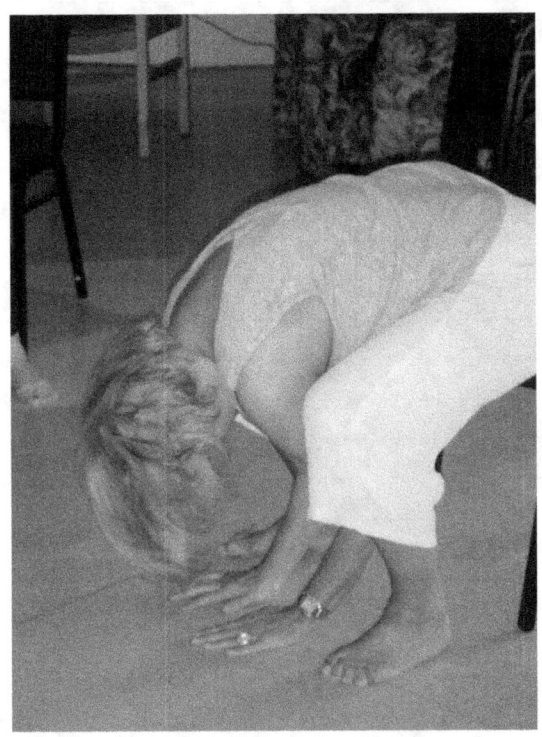

1. Sit on edge of the chair.
2. Spread legs wide apart.
3. Press feet into the floor.
4. *Inhale* and stretch torso upward.
5. Slowly bend forward from the hips as you *exhale.*
6. Hold your elbows on your thighs or place fingertips or hands on the floor.
7. Relax head and neck.
8. Take a few deep breaths.
9. *Exhale* as you slowly sit up.

#6: BOAT - NAVASANA

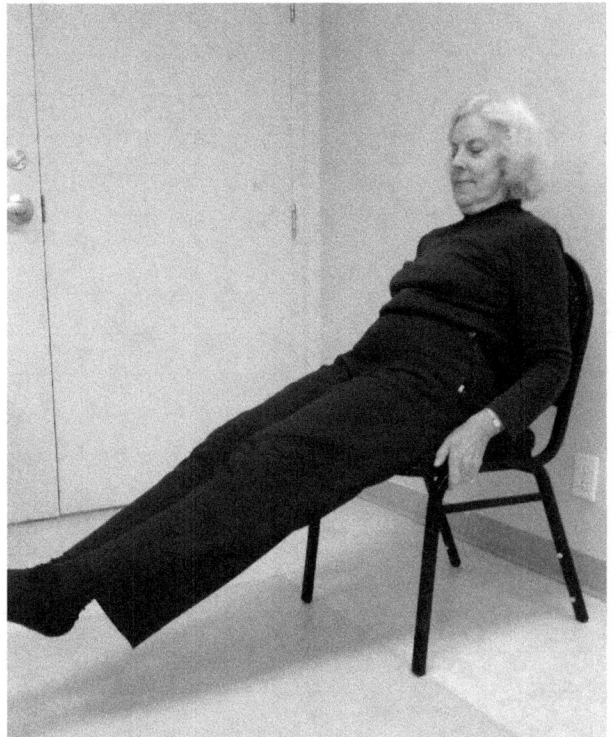

1. *Inhale* and sit tall.
2. Keep your arms relaxed on your thighs or holding the chair sides.
3. *Exhale* and slowly lean back until your back touches the chair back.
4. Stay leaning back as you *inhale* fully.
5. *Exhale* and slowly lift your legs a few inches from the floor.
6. Keep your legs lifted for a few breaths.
7. *Exhale* bringing legs back to the floor.
8. *Inhale* fully then *exhale* to sit up tall.
9. Repeat this movement 3 to 5 times.

#7: KNEE TO NOSE -   PAVANMUKTASANA

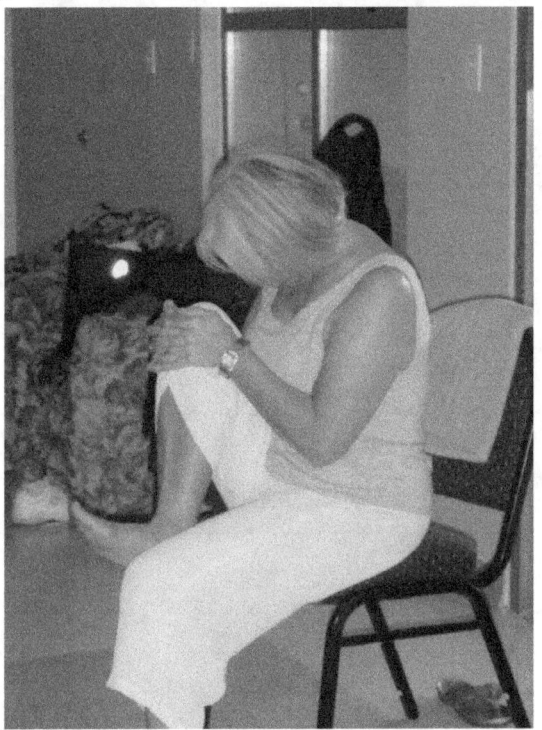

1. *Inhale* and sit tall.
2. *Exhaling* as you slowly raise your knee towards your nose.
3. Interlace your fingers below your knee to bring your leg closer to your body.
4. *Exhale* as you slowly place your foot back on the floor.
5. Repeat with the same leg a few times.
6. Switch legs.

#8: CHAIR TWIST - BHARADHVAJASANA

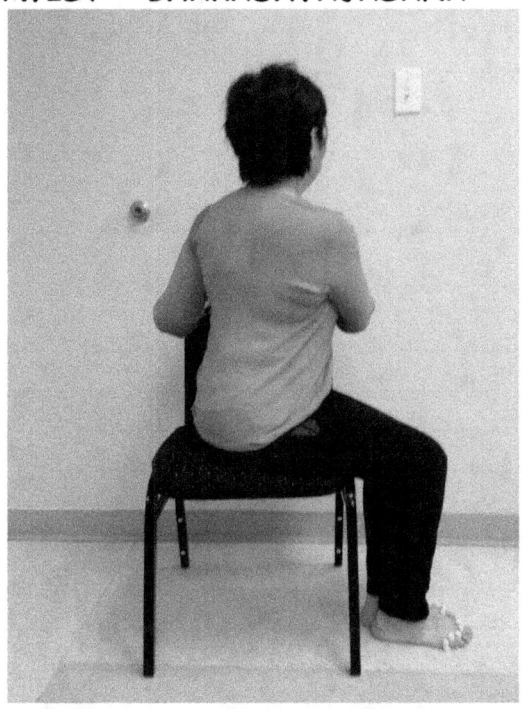

1. Sit sideways on the seat of the chair.
2. Press feet into the floor, lift rib cage out of your hips to lengthen your spine, stretch your shoulders back and down.
3. Keep ankles under your knees and knees two fists apart.
4. *Inhale* as you raise arms straight up, and *exhale* as you turn to grab the chair back.
5. Continue stretching upwards as you twist.
6. Continue twisting for a few more breaths.
7. Turn back as you *exhale.*
8. Move to the opposite side of the chair and repeat on other side.

#9: COBRA - BHUJANGASANA

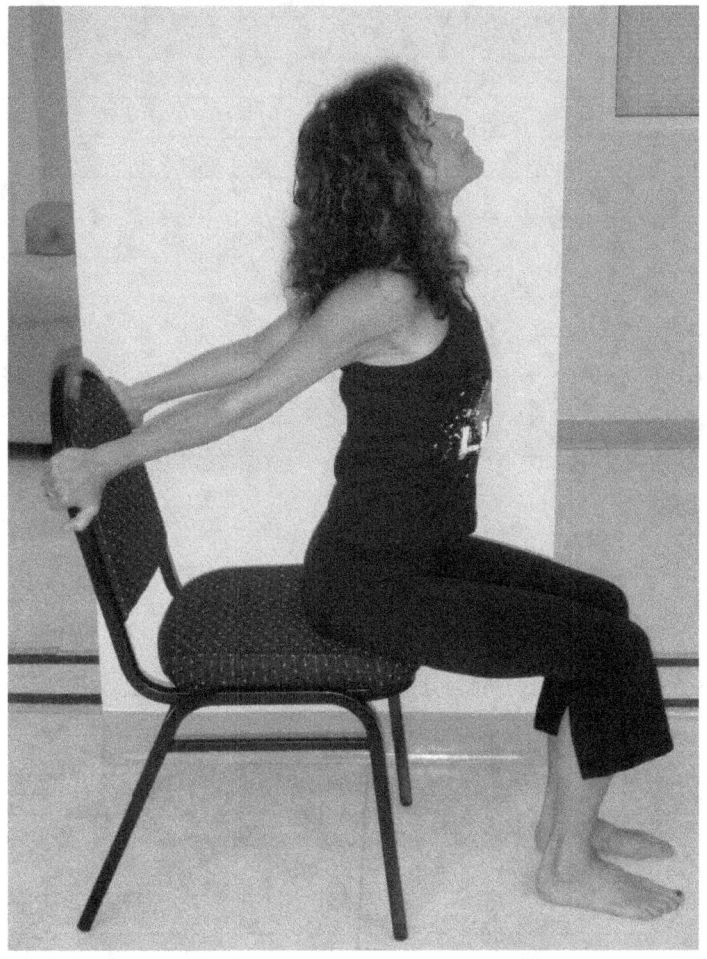

1. Place your hands behind you and firmly grip the sides of the chair.
2. Try to keep your hands straight as you *inhale* and arch your back.
3. Lift your heart up and look up.
4. Stay in this position for a few breaths.
5. *Exhale* to relax.

#10 CONSCIOUS RELAXATION - SAVASANA

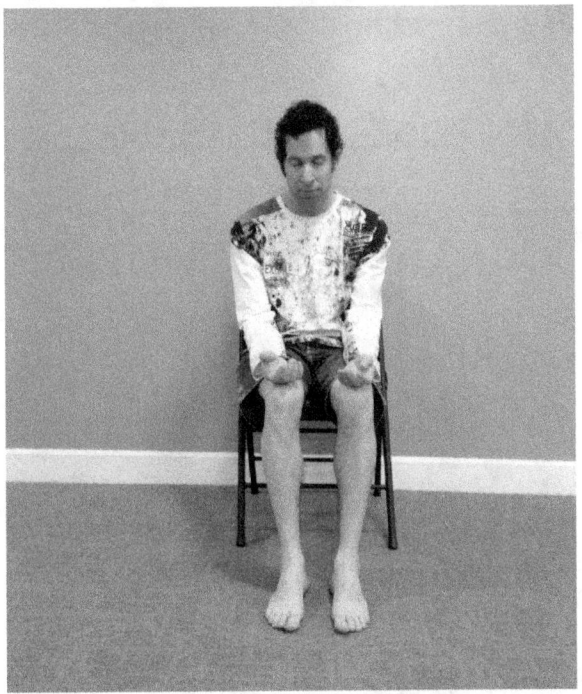

1. Wiggle into a comfortable stillness.
2. Sit still.
3. Focus your closed eyes on the area between your eyebrows or the tip of your nose.
4. Observe your breath, letting your thoughts drift by.
5. Breathe easily and consciously, relaxing your whole body for 3 to 5 minutes.
6. Turn your palms up and recite softly, 10 times, out loud, touching your thumb to each finger "May I Be Happy."
7. Bow your head to your heart and say "Namaste."

ASANAS: POSTURES
SEQUENCE #2 Standing

#1: MOUNTAIN POSE - TADASANA

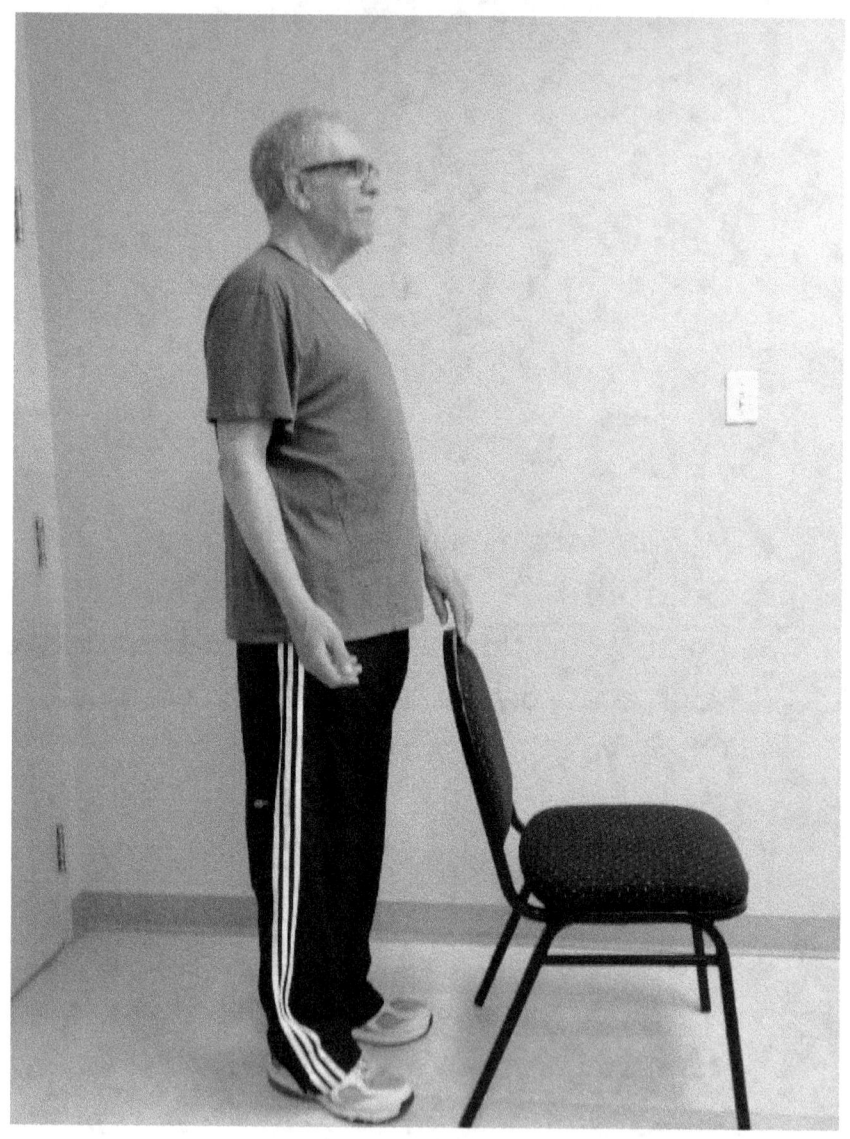

#1: MOUNTAIN POSE - TADASANA

1. Stand with your feet together (or two fists apart).
2. Stretch out your toes and keep them relaxed.
3. Keep your heels parallel and behind your toes.
4. Press your feet firmly down on the floor.
5. Tighten and pull up your kneecaps and quadriceps.
6. Tighten your tush (buttocks).
7. Keep your head upright and look straight ahead.
8. Extend your arms alongside your body with palms facing your thighs and fingers pointing down.
9. Keep head and spine in a straight line.
10. Pull your lower abdomen in and up.
11. Lift your sternum and broaden your chest.
12. Rest most of your weight on your heels.

_____

_____

_____

_____

_____

#2: CAMEL POSE - USTRASANA

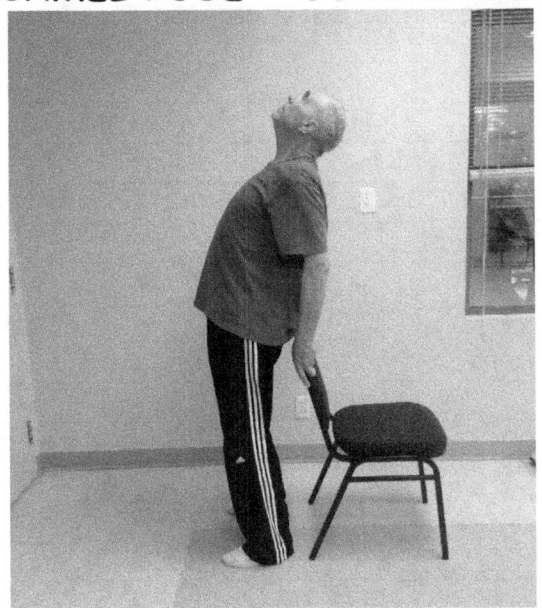

1. Behind your chair, stand tall in Tadasana (Mountain pose).
2. *Inhale* and push your shoulders back.
3. *Exhale* and hold the back of the chair.
4. *Inhale*, slowly lifting and broadening your chest, gently arching your back.
5. Look up and *exhale*.
6. Push down with your feet and feel a lengthening of your spine.
7. Breathe evenly.
8. *Exhale* to bring your body back to an upright position.
9. Release your arms to your side.

#3: CAT - COBRA

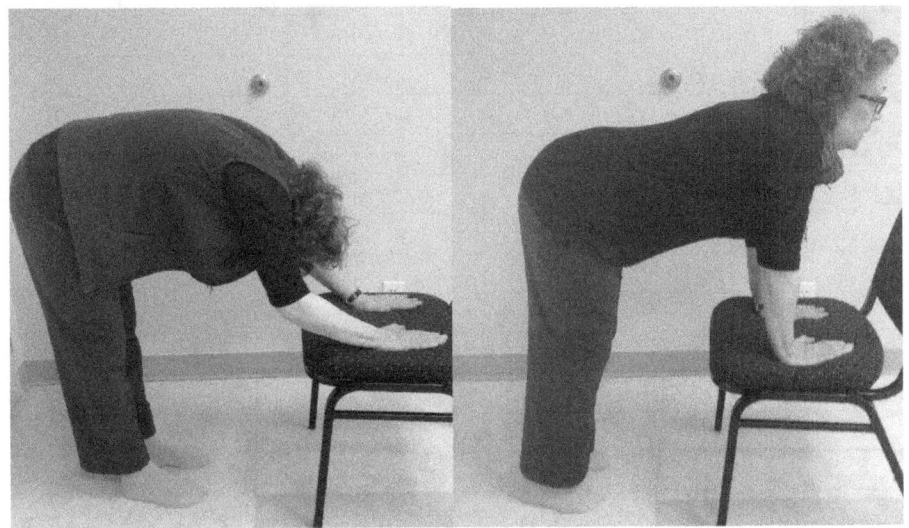

1. Stand in front of the chair seat with feet parallel and apart.
2. *Inhale.*
3. Keep a soft bend in your knees
4. *Exhale* slowly as you bend to place your hands on the seat of the chair.
5. *Inhale* as you slowly arch your back, raising your head and your hips.
6. As you *exhale* round your back, keeping your arms straight.
7. Try to hold your stomach muscles in.
8. Repeat a few times breathing slowly, evenly and deeply.
9. *Exhale* to slowly stand up.

#4: FORWARD FOLD - UTTANASANA

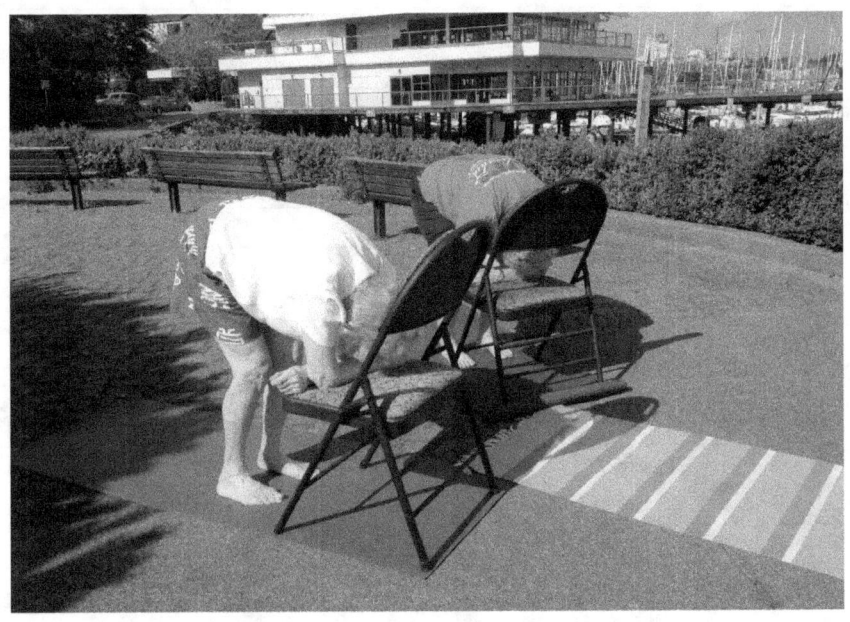

1. Stand tall in Tadasana (mountain pose).
2. Press feet into the floor.
3. Bend your knees slightly.
4. *Inhale* and stretch torso upward as you raise your arms.
5. Slowly bend forward from the hips as you *exhale.*
6. Place your elbows on the seat of the chair.
7. Relax head and neck.
8. Take a few breaths.
9. *Exhale* as you slowly stand up.

#5: HALF MOON

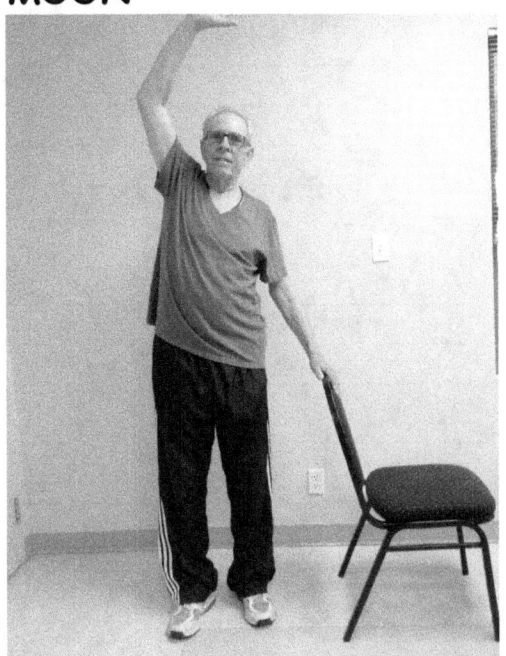

1. Stand up straight, behind your chair. Feet are hip distance apart.
2. Hold the back of chair with left hand.
3. As you *inhale*, slowly raise your outstretched right arm up over your head.
4. As you *exhale*, gently lean your upper body to the left.
5. *Inhale* and slowly stand up straight again
6. Repeat a few times.
7. On the last inhalation, keep erect and as you *exhale*, slowly lower your right arm.
8. Repeat this movement with the right arm holding the back of the chair.

#6: FLAT BACK - ARDHA UTTANASANA

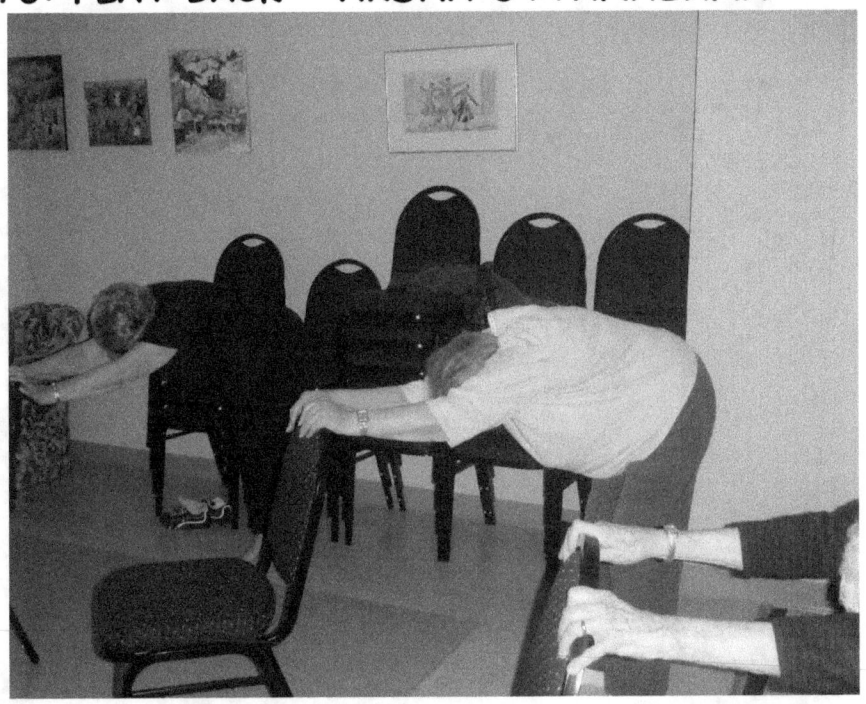

1. Stand at an appropriate distance from the chair back.
2. Stretch your arms up, then bend forward
3. Place your hands to hold the back of the chair.
4. Move your thighs back and stretch your trunk forward with knees slightly bent.
5. Try to keep your arms straight.
6. Breathe gently and evenly.
7. *Inhale* as you slowly step towards the chair back.
8. *Exhale* as you slowly stand up.

#7: CHAIR POSE-UTKATASANA

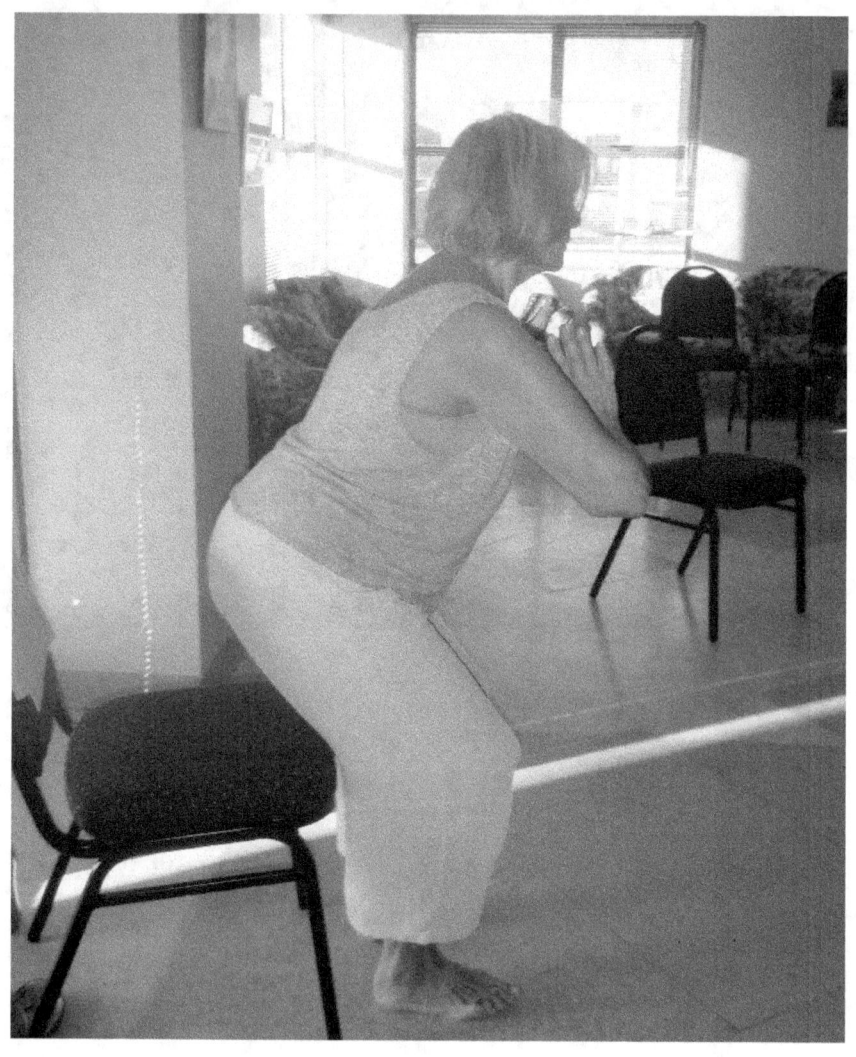

#7: CHAIR POSE-UTKATASANA

1. Stand in Tadasana (mountain pose).
2. *Inhale* and raise your arms up over your head.
3. Lengthen your spine without arching the lower back.
4. Keep palms facing each other (or prayer hands variation).
5. *Exhale* and bend your knees as though you were sitting in a chair.
6. Try to keep thighs parallel to each other.
7. Drop tailbone down, and lift lower belly in and up, looking straight ahead.
8. Sink your weight into your heels.
9. Keep shoulders down away from ears.
10. Hold the posture and breathe.
11. *Inhale* and straighten your legs.
12. *Exhale* and release your arms to your sides.

_____
_____
_____
_____
_____
_____
_____
_____
_____
_____

#8: THE STORK-BAKA ASANA

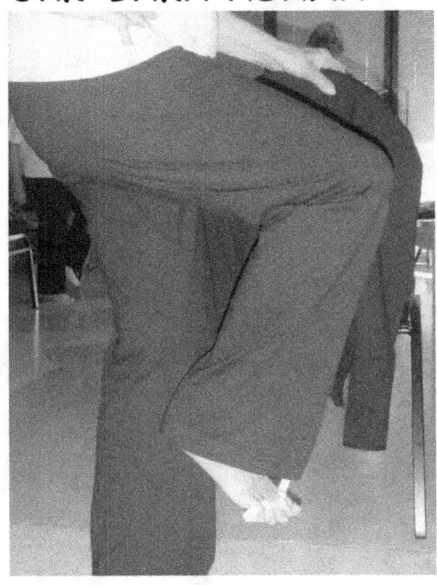

1. Stand up tall and hold on to the chair with left hand.
2. *Inhale* as you slowly lift right leg directly in front of you.
3. Bend your knee without bending the hips or waste area.
4. Keep toes flexed.
5. Lift as high as possible towards your chest
6. *Exhale* as you slowly lower your leg.
7. Pause, breathing fully.
8. Repeat movement with same leg a few times.
9. Change to hold chair with right hand, lifting left leg.

#9: TREE-VRIKSHASANA

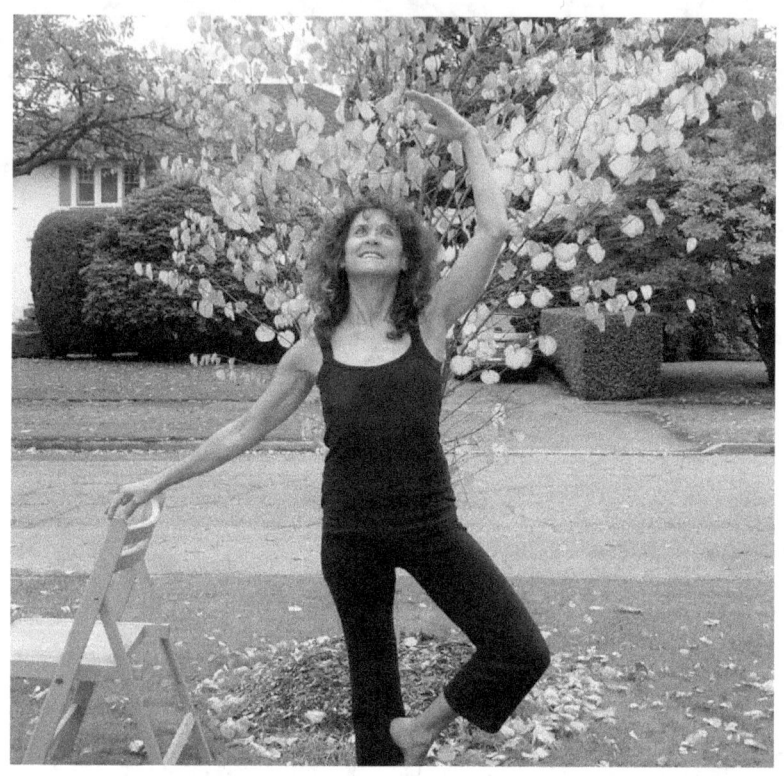

_____
_____
_____
_____
_____
_____
_____
_____
_____
_____
_____
_____
_____

#9: TREE-VRIKSHASANA

1. Stand in Tadasana holding on to the chair with right hand.
2. Shift weight into right foot pressing evenly and firmly into the floor.
3. Bend left knee and place the sole against the inner calf.
4. Toes point towards the floor.
5. Press the left foot into the right leg with equal pressure.
6. Lengthen tailbone towards the floor
7. Find your drishti (focus point) and gaze softly.
8. When steady raise your left arm over your head.
9. Reach entire body upward and breathe evenly.
10. Relax shoulders, neck and face.
11. With an *exhalation*, step back to Tadasana.
12. Repeat on other side.

#10: HAMSTRING STRETCH-PADANGUSTHASANA

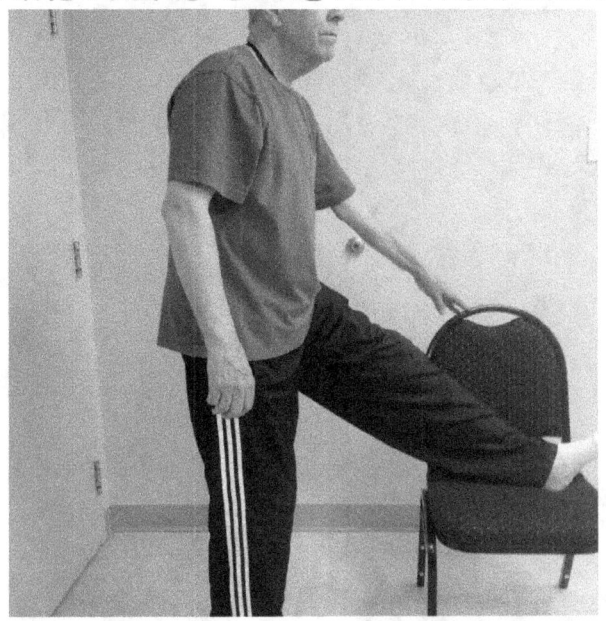

1. Stand facing the right side of your chair.
2. Hold on to the chair back with your left hand.
3. Shift your weight to your right foot.
4. With an *exhale* lift left knee and place heel onto the seat.
5. Try to straighten your leg.
6. Flex your toes and *inhale*.
7. Leading with your heart, *exhale* and slowly lean over your straightened leg.
8. Relax in this position for a few breaths.
9. On an *exhale* slowly raise your body up.
10. On the next *exhale*, bring your right leg to the floor.
11. Repeat with other leg.

#11: WARRIOR I-VIRABHADRASANA I

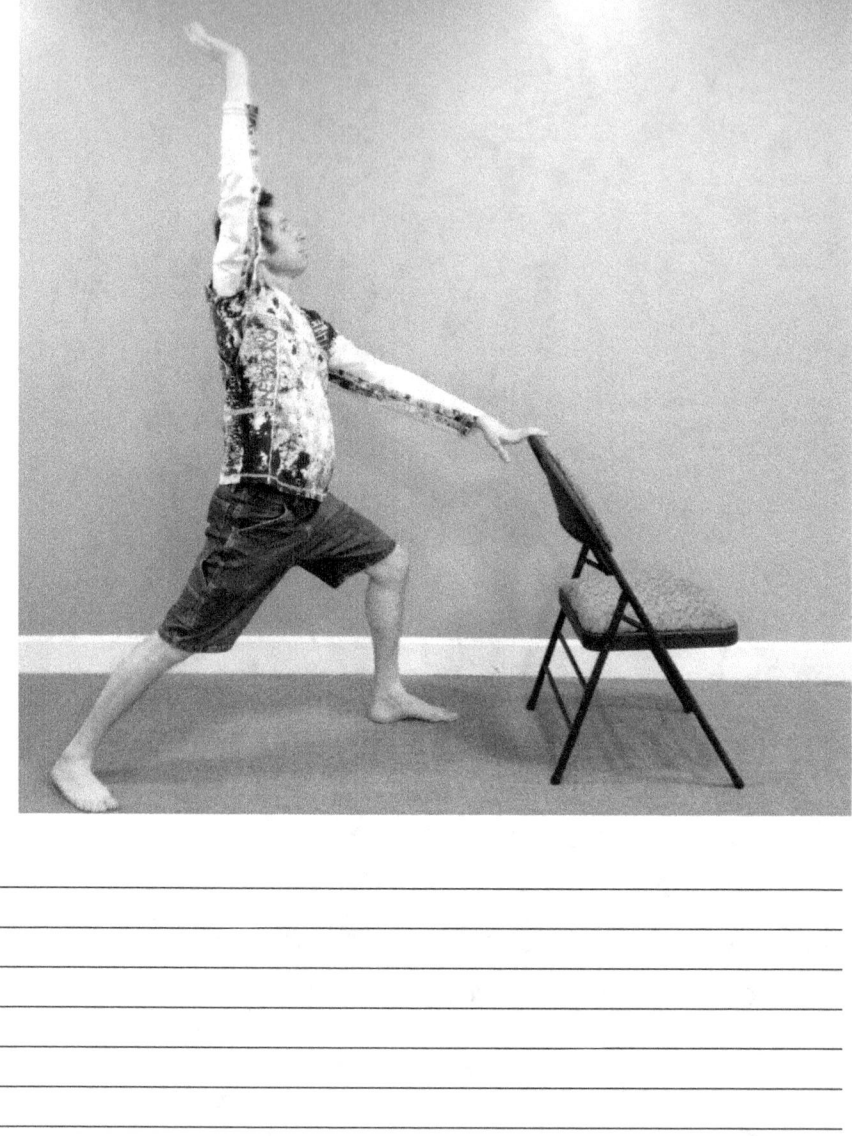

_____

_____

_____

_____

_____

_____

_____

_____

_____

_____

_____

#11: WARRIOR I-VIRABHADRASANA I

1. Stand in Tadasana behind the chair.
2. Hold on to the chair with left hand.
3. Step right foot back one leg length.
4. Left foot faces forward, right foot turned out slightly to 45 degrees.
5. Keep your trunk and hips facing forward.
6. *Exhale* and bend left leg keeping the knee directly over the ankle.
7. *Inhale* and raise your right hand keeping palm facing in.
8. Ground down through the back foot.
9. Keep head in a neutral position or tilt it back to gaze up.
10. Hold the pose and take a few breaths.
11. *Inhale* and straighten left leg, stepping back to Tadasana. Repeat on other side.

#12: WARRIOR II-VIRABHADRASANA II

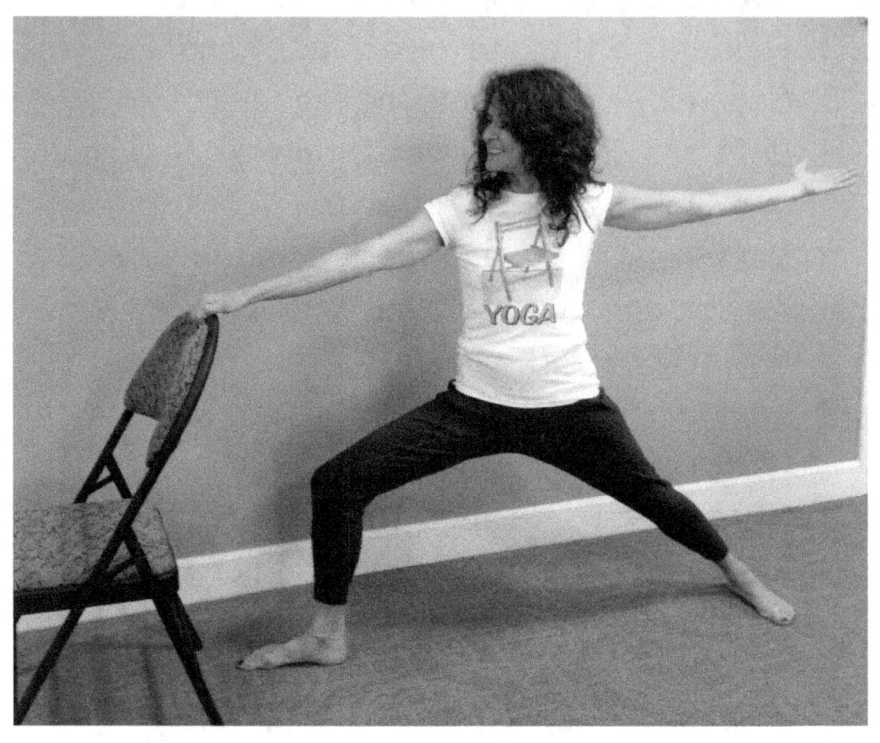

_____
_____
_____
_____
_____
_____
_____
_____
_____
_____
_____
_____

#12: WARRIOR II-VIRABHADRASANA II

1. Stand in Tadasana behind your chair.
2. Hold on to the chair with right hand.
3. *Exhale* and step left foot back about three to four feet.
4. Place left foot slightly turned inwards, right foot pointing straight forward.
5. Left foot directly behind heel of front foot.
6. Hips bones are level and turned sideways.
7. *Exhale* and bend the right knee so that it is directly over the ankle.
8. Keep left heel pressed firmly into the floor and right knee pointing forward.
9. Drop tailbone and engage abdomen.
10. Centre weight between legs and rib cage over pelvis.
11. Raise left arm up to shoulder level, palm facing down.
12. Stretch sideways keeping shoulder relaxed.
13. Gaze out past middle finger of right hand.
14. *Inhale* and straighten right knee, lower arm.
15. *Exhale* coming back to Tadasana. Now the other side.

#13: CONSCIOUS RELAXATION-SAVASANA

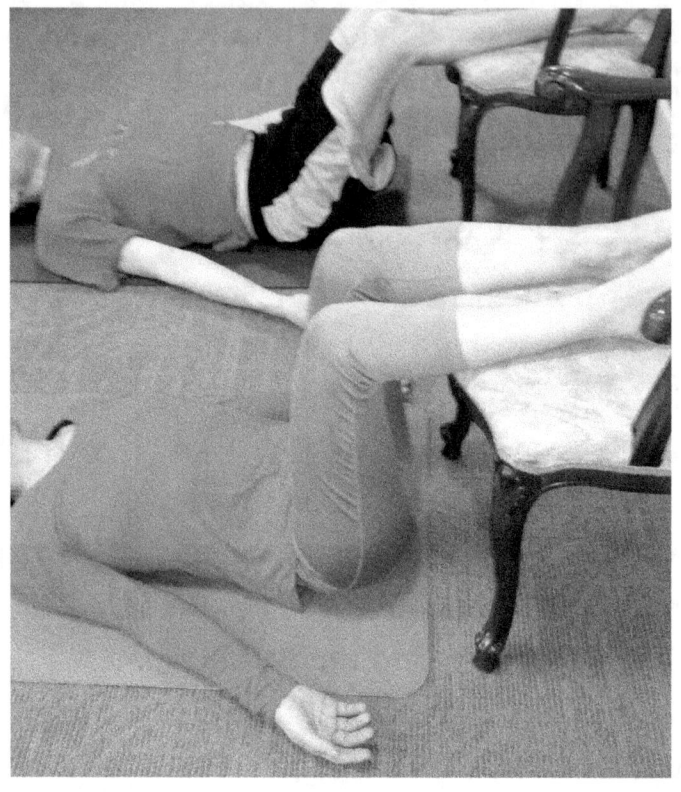

#13: CONSCIOUS RELAXATION-SAVASANA

1. Lay down on back.
2. Lift legs onto seat of chair with knees bent.
3. Stretch arms out to sides slightly away from body, palms up.
4. Make sure shoulder blades are resting evenly on the floor.
5. Release tension in neck and shoulders
6. Let the body become heavy, sinking into the floor.
7. Soften the jaw, eyes and face
8. Focus closed eyes between eyebrows.
9. Stay in this pose a minimum of 5 minutes.
10. To come out slowly wiggle fingers and toes.
11. Lifting legs off the chair, roll to right side in a fetal position, before slowly coming up to sitting.

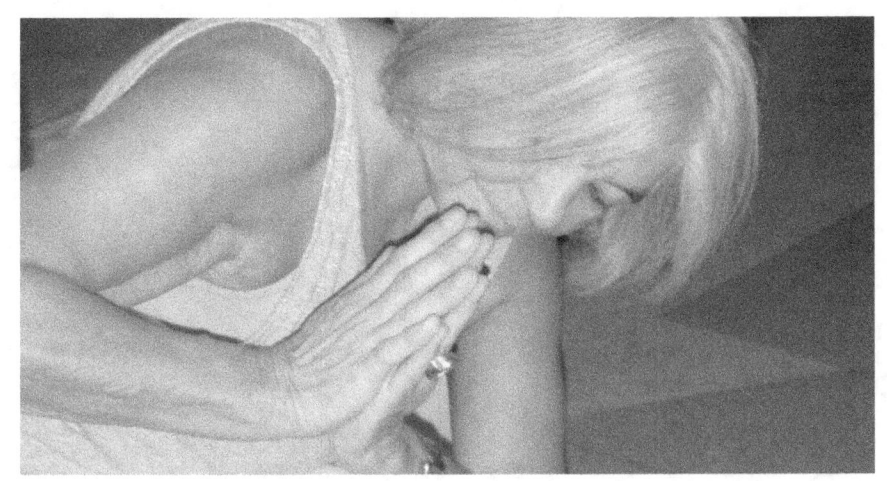

NAMASTE

FROM
MY HEART TO YOURS

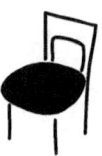

ABOUT ANNETTE WERTMANN

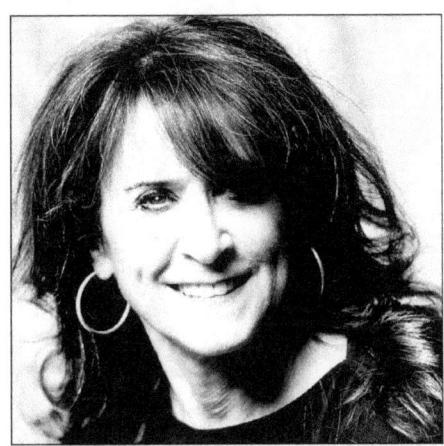

Annette Wertman is a certified yoga instructor and registered music therapist. She recently received an M.A. in Gerontology from Simon Fraser University. The highlight report of her thesis on *Yoga and Older Adults* is available on her website, http://agelessyoga.ca.

Annette teaches "Yoga with a Chair" or "Chair Yoga" throughout greater Vancouver, British Columbia, Canada. She has also presented workshops at the Vancouver Yoga Show, the Toronto Yoga Show, the Canadian Association of Gerontology, the Canadian Nurses Association, the International Council on Active Aging, the Council of Senior Citizens' Organizations of BC and BC Recreation and Parks Board. She offers Chair Yoga Teacher Training through Semperviva Yoga School in Vancouver.

For more information about Annette, visit her website, **http://agelessyoga.ca** or contact her at annette@agelessyoga.ca to book a speech, workshop or therapy session.

www.ingramcontent.com/pod-product-compliance
Lightning Source LLC
Chambersburg PA
CBHW060225290526
45789CB00003B/1417